Teens and Sex

How Should We Teach Them?

Paul David Tripp

P&R
PUBLISHING
P.O. BOX 817 • PHILLIPSBURG • NEW JERSEY 08865-0817

It doesn't take much insight to be concerned about the culture in which our children are growing. Our children are being powerfully influenced by an unbiblical view of life, particularly in the area of sexuality. This lie is being peddled to our children incessantly, from the teen magazines that portray a distorted sexuality to the overtly sexual images of MTV music videos. As Christian parents, we need to be teaching our children the life-transforming truths that expose the counterfeits for what they are. And we must present these truths in a way that is understandable to the average young person. To do that, we must be sure that we as parents are thinking in a genuinely biblical way about teenagers and sexuality. That challenge is the focus of this booklet.

The State of the Culture: Institutionalizing Sexual Idolatry

The overt sexual expression in our culture should not surprise us since it is rooted in a view of life that has exchanged the worship and service of the Creator for the worship and service of the created thing (see Rom. 1:21–25). This view of life holds these "truths" to be self-evident:

1. People are *ultimate* and *autonomous*. That is, there is nothing more important than the individual. I am free from any authority I do not choose to follow.
2. The highest human value and experience is personal satisfaction and pleasure.
3. I must be constantly vigilant that my "needs" are met.
4. The most important love is the love of self.
5. With pleasure, bigger is better. There is a constant desire for greater stimulation.
6. The here and now is what is important. There is a constant pursuit of instant gratification.
7. The physical person is more important than the spiritual person.

In a culture that looks at people as ultimate, God as absent, and pleasure as the highest experience, it is no wonder that sexuality becomes such a dominant force. It provides a powerful pathway to instant physical pleasure. It provides false worship (counterfeiting the first great command) and false relationship (counterfeiting the second great command). Every institution in our culture is infected with a distorted view of human sexuality. This being so, our children need us to be radically active in countering it.

The State of the Church: Giving Mixed Messages to Our Teens

Unfortunately, our ability to counter distorted views is hindered by what I see as the church's ambivalence about sex. We need to face the ways this ambivalence has affected our teenagers.

Here is what I mean: As Christians, we say that sex is a wonderful gift from God, yet we are strangely silent on the topic and uncomfortable in the rare instances when it is discussed. This leads to a lack of sexual balance, a lack of sexual openness, and a lack of clear, practical sexual education. Sex tends to get placed outside the boundaries of the normative Christian worldview.

Is it surprising, then, that the typical teenager assumes that Christianity is "sex-negative"? That is, basically *against* sex? The church has been perceived this way for a long time, and it is surely the perception of many teens today.

I can remember taking my nine- and eleven-year-old sons out for pizza to talk to them about sex. After we ordered I opened up the subject, took out a pen and began drawing on a napkin. At first my sons were surprised that I was willing to talk with such openness. Then they figured that if I was not embarrassed to talk with them about sex, they should not be either. My goal was to treat this area in the same way I had treated other areas—as an important piece of the Christian world-and-life view that I was seeking to instill in them. I had every reason to discuss the subject and no reason to be embarrassed or silent.

Why are we as Christians so ambivalent about sex? Why do we tend to give confusing signals to our teens? It seems that this ambivalence is rooted in three biblical misunderstandings:

1. The church has tended to view sexuality as less than good and godly.

2. We have tended to view sin as behavioral and physical, rather than a matter of the heart.
3. We have tended to view teenage choice and behavior as biologically determined.

If the church unwittingly implies that it is "sex-negative," it loses its authority to guide the teenager's sexual life. Teens won't come to the Christian community with their sexual questions, fears, and experiences. They are left with one of three options. (1) They can try to live with the church's embarrassed silence and cope with their questions, interests, and experiences alone. (2) They can assume that Christians do not have sexual questions or problems, and begin to question their own relationship with the Lord when they do. (3) They can go where information and open discussion are readily available—that is, the world. Here they will be able to ask their questions and get answers, no matter how regrettable they may be.

We cannot live with the ambivalence of the church and allow the world to guide our teens in this or any other area. The Christian community, from the home to the organized church, must be prepared to act, to educate, to guide, and to restore. Later, I will lay out a practical agenda for dealing with teens in the area of sex.

A Biblical View of Teenagers

One major reason the church has been ineffective in dealing with our teens in this area is that we have bought into an unbiblical view of adolescence. I heard it expressed recently at a conference. "We just have to expect our teenagers to be rebellious; all of us were. We just need to ride it out," a father said. His wife chimed in, "You can't argue with hormones!" This is the view of most Christian parents as they view the teenage years. The question is, Is this a biblical view?

Too often, when it comes to teenagers, we have bought into a biological model of behavior. We talk about our teenagers as collections of raging, rebel hormones encased in developing skin. We see our goal as somehow chaining those hormones so that we all can survive until they reach age twenty. Many parents who talk to me about their teens talk without hope because they see them as victims of biological urges that drive them to do crazy things. It is implied that for this age span, Scripture doesn't work, the gospel doesn't work, talking doesn't work. But we cannot be satisfied with this view of teenagers. As in all other areas of life, we need a view that is distinctly biblical.

In 2 Timothy 2:22, Paul exhorts Timothy to "flee the evil desires [lusts] of youth." This interesting phrase speaks to the way we view teenagers and the teen years. First, notice that the Bible is not naive about this time of life. There are lusts that uniquely plague youth, particularly powerful temptations that need to be faced. Scripture is urging us to ask the question, What evil desires can grip a person during this phase of life?

Another thing that can be drawn from Paul's qualifier, "youthful" (KJV), is that *each* phase of life has its own set of temptations. The temptations of the young man and the old man are not totally different, yet they are not identical. Paul is reminding Timothy to be aware of who he is and where the pockets of temptation exist around him.

Another thing that can be drawn from this phrase is that teenagers have not been singled out for particular sacrifice and suffering. Each person at each time in his life, if he seeks to please the Lord, must watch, pray, stand fast, and fight lest he fall into temptation. The young person is called to run from the evil desires of youth, while the older person is called to guard against the temptations unique to age. Each person must accept each stage of warfare in the normal Christian life.

In the first seven chapters of the book of Proverbs, a father addresses his son, detailing what it means to live wisely and foolishly. He warns his son about the particular temptations of his youth. This portion of Scripture establishes a model of teenage struggles that contrasts with the current biological model. We can identify five characteristics of young people from these chapters:

1. Teenagers don't tend to value wisdom. My teenagers don't come to me at the end of the day and say, "Boy, Dad, I've been thinking, and I realize that I have an abject lack of wisdom. Can I sit at your feet and glean the wisdom you have received from your years of walking with the Lord?" Most of us would be shocked at such a thing!

Teenagers tend to be closed. They tend to be defensive. They don't love correction or long for wisdom and understanding. Teenagers tend to be externally focused, more concerned about physical things than spiritual things. So the father in Proverbs says to his son many times and in many ways, "Get wisdom!"

2. Young people tend to be unwise in their choice of companions. What parent hasn't winced as their teenager has brought home his latest, greatest friend who looks like a prison escapee! The parent struggles to be polite while thinking, "I don't want you to ever see this person again!"

Teenagers tend to be unwise in choosing those who influence their lives. And they tend to get easily hurt if you criticize their friends.

3. Teenagers don't tend to focus on the heart. In the middle of this section of Proverbs the author says, "Above all else, guard your heart, for it is the wellspring of life" (4:23). He is telling his son that the heart needs to be the focus of his concern, though it is the very thing teenagers most easily ignore.

As a father, I want to make my children aware of the issues of their hearts. That is not what my children are interested in naturally. As sinners, they bring a natural legalism to our relationship. They want to know what the rule is and how close they can get to the boundaries without getting in trouble. They want to know what will happen if they actually cross the boundaries. Their view of God's law is the exact opposite of what Christ expressed in the Sermon on the Mount (Matt. 5:17–48). Teenagers tend to focus on the letter of the law and not the spirit. If we are unaware of this and ignore the heart that lies beneath the behavior, we may be encouraging the kind of pharisaism that Christ is confronting in his sermon. We may be raising children who "honor [God] with their lips, but their hearts are far from [him]" (Matt. 15:8).

4. Young people don't tend to have an eschatological perspective. The view of life that brings godly responsibility to one's sexuality is rooted in eternity, but for the teenager eternity is distant and irrelevant. Teens are experts in instant gratification, not long-term outcomes. Thus, the message of the Proverbs father to his son is, "Remember, son, this is not all there is. Don't let the desires of the moment trick you into forgetting what is to come. The seeds you plant now you will harvest later."

5. Teenagers tend to be uniquely suscep-tible to sexual temptation. No issue gets more attention in this Scripture portion than this one. Proverbs 5 and 7 are entirely dedicated to this issue. During the teen years, our children see and feel things that they never have before, yet they often lack the maturity to deal with those experiences in a godly fashion.

These five characteristics remind us of what the teenager brings to moments of sexual temptation. Honestly examining them should remind us not of how utterly different teenagers are but of how much they are like us. Each of us can relate to being blind to issues of the heart, to living for the moment, to reject-ing wisdom and correction. These are issues of the fallen nature, not just a particular phase of life. At that level we can humbly bring the hope of the gospel to our teenagers instead of the harsh judgment that comes when we forget who *we* are.

A Biblical Model of Sexuality

What is it that we want our teenagers to understand about their sexuality? Four things are critical to a Christian model.

Sex Is a Key Way a Person Expresses Worship (Rom. 1:18–27)

Romans 1:21–27 portrays sex as a principal way in which a person reveals what is really ruling his life. Sexual sin is by its very nature idolatrous; that is, it is a place where we refuse to live for God's glory. It is driven by the sinful desires of the heart rather than a desire to live by God's principles for his pleasure. A person submits his heart and body to God's higher agenda or uses them to get pleasure when and where he wishes. Here a person exchanges the protection and freedom of God's truth for a host of self-serving lies.

Our teens need to see life as worship. They are either living in covenant with God, hoping in his promises, obeying his commands, relying on his grace, and desiring his glory, or they are living in an idol covenant where some part of creation has replaced the Creator, and they live for personal pleasure and the glory of self.

Sadly, few parents or youth leaders have conversations with teenagers on this level. In the absence of this critical perspective, Scripture is seen as a fire escape for the future and a list of *dos* and *don'ts* for the present. The Christian life is reduced to a pharisaical "do this and please Jesus" religion.

Sex Is a Key Way a Person Expresses His Identity (1 Cor. 6:12–20)

In the final analysis, human beings live out one of only two identities: that I am ultimate and autonomous or that I am created and dependent on God. The question underlying all human thought, motive, and behavior is, Will I live out my identity as a creature of God (and for the believer, as a child of God) or will I live as my own god with no higher agenda than my own satisfaction?

In 1 Corinthians 6 Paul roots his entire discussion of sexual immorality in the identity of the believer. He points out four aspects of the Christian's identity that provide wonderful boundaries for sex and every area of life:

1. I am a servant of Christ. " 'Everything is permissible for me'—but I will not be mastered by anything" (v. 12). Christ has freed his children from bondage to the cravings of the sinful nature, not to self-centered "liberty" but to the wonderful freedom found only as they accept their slavery to him (see Rom. 6:1–14). Our sexual lives will express either a joyful submission to Christ or an allegiance to another master.

2. I am an eternal being. "By his power God raised the Lord from the dead, and he will raise us also" (1 Cor. 6:14). This world is not all there is; neither its sufferings nor its pleasures are worth comparing to the glory that is to come. A future hope changes the way a believer looks at the pressures, opportunities, and responsibilities of the moment. She lives patiently, conscious of the eternal value of every sacrifice she makes.

3. I am one with Christ. "Do you not know that your bodies are members of Christ himself? . . . He who unites himself with the Lord is one with him in spirit" (vv. 15, 17). Believers are actually joined to Christ in an inseparable union. Since our spirits are one with him, our bodies belong to Christ as well, so that our lives would practically express the will of Christ. Independence is a delusion.

4. I am the property of Christ. "You are not your own; you were bought at a price. Therefore honor God with your body" (vv. 19–20). God bought us when he paid the price with the blood of his Son. We belong to him. We do not belong to ourselves! Peter says that we are "a people for God's own possession" (1 Peter 2:9 NASB). Our obligation—and joy—is to please our Owner.

Do you see how a biblical sense of identity can be a powerful defense against "youthful lusts"? Unfortunately, few people working with teens address the problem at this level. But unless we do, teens will buy into the world's definitions of identity, in which biblical morality and the worshipful sacrifices it demands no longer make any sense. This is why, as parents, we need a bigger goal than keeping our teens "out of trouble." We should settle for nothing less than their becoming "partakers of [his] divine nature" (2 Peter 1:4 KJV).

Sex Is a Key Revealer of a Person's Heart (Eph. 5:3–7)

In the Sermon on the Mount, Christ declares that it is not enough to say, "I have not physically committed adultery; therefore, I am pure." For Christ, *lust* breaks the command against adultery. Another way of saying this is that a person's sexual behavior is a key revealer of what is ruling her heart. This is why a rejection of God's revelation and authority leads to all kinds of sexual sin. Paul states it very plainly in Ephesians 5: The sexually immoral person is an idolater in the thoughts, motives, desires, demands, expectations, treasures, or idols of his heart. For that reason, it is not enough to try to keep our teens out of trouble if by that we mean keeping them from outward, physical sin. We must help our teens face the heart sins that physical sexual sin reveals.

Sex Is a Key Revealer of My Need of Grace (Rom. 7:7–25)

Sex confronts me with my inability. In light of God's standard of absolute purity, I say with Paul, "I know that nothing good lives in me, that is, in my sinful nature" (7:18). My utter inability to meet God's standard confronts me also with the reality and majesty of his grace. "Where sin increased, grace increased all the more" (5:20). I can no more fulfill God's call to sexual purity in my own strength than I can save myself.

Our young people need to connect their sexual struggles to these larger gospel themes. When they do, they will not only find victory, but they can develop a new dependency on Jesus and a deeper love for him. The lies of self-sufficiency and self-righteousness are exposed, giving us an opportunity to bring teens the hope of the gospel in ways they have never before grasped.

Establish Biblical Goals for Teens and Sex

There has been a renewed interest in virginity both inside and outside the church. Christian and community groups are rallying teenagers to sign abstinence contracts, committing themselves to virginity until marriage. I, too, want my children to abstain from sexual intercourse until marriage, but this agenda does not go far enough.

For one thing, it moves us toward a less-than-biblical definition of moral purity. To be physically abstinent is not the same as being morally pure! Moral purity is a matter of the heart. If the heart is not pure, the body will not be kept pure for long. God wants nothing less than the hearts of his people (Ezek. 14:5). We cannot allow our teens to relax because they have kept the letter of the law while breaking the spirit, like the scribes and Pharisees (Matt. 5:17–20).

A second problem is that the abstinence agenda can skew an evaluation of our teenagers' relationships with the opposite sex. Is a physically abstinent relationship automatically God-honoring? A person could have a constellation of idolatrous goals for a relationship and yet be physically abstinent. We don't want our teens to be comfortable with self-centered, manipulative friendships simply because they do not include intercourse.

Let me demonstrate the shallowness of the abstinence goal. If you set abstinence as the standard for any other relationship, it would make no sense at all. For example, just because I don't have sexual relations with my children does not mean that my relationship with them is healthy and all that God has designed it to be! The physical abstinence issue is so obvious here that it is not even a primary standard for evaluating parent-child relationships. The same should be true in the case of teen relationships. Abstinence is at most a starting point from which to assess our children's friendships biblically.

Positively, what we are dealing with are boundary issues. In sexual matters, where do we set the boundaries for our children? In

Matthew 5:27–30, Christ charges that the teachers of the law put the boundaries of sexual purity in the wrong place, at the edge of behavior, misunderstanding the law's intent. Christ placed the boundaries squarely within the *heart*. This was the original intent of the law.

We must place the boundaries where Christ does. Keeping within the physical boundaries is not a high enough goal. Our goal should be to live within the heart boundaries and not settle for culturally popular, humanly doable goals that encourage self-righteousness without solving the problem. We must uphold God's standards and watch his Spirit recapture the hearts of our children.

A Threefold Plan for Helping Teens

There are three ways in which we want to communicate these biblical principles about sex to our teenagers.

Prevention: Responsibly Educating Our Teens

As we have seen, it is important to give teens a full biblical perspective as the foundation for a practical sexual agenda. I stress the following principles in my work with teenagers:

1. God is the Creator, and it is important to understand his original purpose for all things (Ps. 24).

2. People are God's creatures, and therefore we are responsible to him for all we are and do. The goal of life is to live for his pleasure and glory (Gen. 1; Col. 3:17).

3. People are unified beings. Sin is both spiritual and physical, a matter of the heart *and* behavior (Rom. 8:1–17).

4. Life is worship. Everything I do expresses worship to God or something else. The deepest questions of human life are not questions of my pain or pleasure, but of what I worship. This is what really determines my approach to life (Rom. 1:18–32).

5. God's way, no matter how hard, is always best. As the psalmist says, all the ways of the Lord are right and true, while the way that seems right to a man leads to death. I will not always

understand *how* God's way is best.
That is why I need a heart of humble
submission to his commands and a
humble faith in his promises (Ps.
19:7–11).

6. Because the goal of life is to follow the
will of God and to live to his glory, I always have a higher agenda than mo-
mentary personal pleasure (see 1 Cor.
6:18–20; Titus 2:9–10).

7. Jesus Christ came not only to protect
us from external evil, but to free us
from slavery to the desires of our sinful
nature, so that we may live under the
control of the Spirit (Eph. 2:1–5; 2 Peter 1:4).

The practical implications for teen sexuality include the following:

1. God does not single out teenagers for
sacrifice and suffering. Rather, he calls
them to experience the joys and bless-
ings found by serving him in everyday
situations.

2. Since God, as Creator, formed our bodies and created sexuality, we will never

properly experience this part of life until we understand his plan and purpose.

3. God's plan is that we would, within his boundaries, enjoy this area without ambivalence or shame.

4. We are unified beings, so our sexuality is never isolated from the other parts of us. Sex is never just a physical act; it is always a matter of the heart. It is not enough to ask whether a person has "had sex" yet. We should also be asking about the desires, motives, and thoughts that shape his or her approach to a relationship.

5. We must always examine the thoughts and motives of our hearts in the area of sex: "Have I accepted the sexual lies and the idols of the culture around me?"

6. A person's approach to sexuality must always be shaped by the Two Great Commands, to love God first and to love our neighbor as ourselves.

Restoration: Counseling Teens Who Have Misused Sex

For teens who have fallen into sexual sin, I suggest this step-by-step counseling plan.

1. Establish a commitment to honesty and accountability. The entire counseling process will fall apart without it.
2. Don't be embarrassed to do careful and specific data gathering. Make sure you know what you are dealing with; don't make unwarranted assumptions.
3. Always move toward issues of the heart. Don't focus only on the shocking behavior and its consequences. Deal with root issues as well.
4. Identify the voices in the teen's life. Who is influencing this teenager? What are they saying? How much has this teenager embraced these perspectives?
5. Call the teenager to biblical repentance (Joel 2:12ff.) that includes the "rending" of the heart. Where has the truth of God been exchanged for a lie? Where has the worship and service of God been exchanged for the worship and service of something else? Lead the teenager through the following steps of repentance:
   * *Consideration:* A willingness to look at my sexual life in the light of Scripture.

- *Confession:* Taking responsibility for my sexual sin before God and resting in his forgiveness.
- *Commitment:* A determination, in the strength God gives, to live a new life in the area of sex.
- *Change:* An identification of changes that will conform my sexual life to God's will, and plans to bring about those changes.

6. Identify places of ongoing temptation and make plans to deal with it.

7. Teach the teenager biblical friendship. Explain God's plan for relationships and encourage the teen to keep the Two Great Commands in each relationship.

8. When restoring a teenager who has been involved in sexual sin, avoid comfortable generalities. Be direct, concrete, and specific in your questions and counsel.

9. Make your agenda a balanced "put off" and "put on" (Eph. 4:22–24). In the area of sex, we often emphasize the "put off" aspect ("Don't have sex") without giving the teen a positive "put

on" agenda. What are some practical, godly goals for the teen's relationships with the opposite sex?

Strategizing: Helping Teens Plan for Godly Relationships

In the face of the conflicting messages teens receive, we need to offer a clear understanding of God's will for their relationships and show how those principles apply to their daily lives. Your efforts would include the following:

1. Give teens a biblical view of relationships that leads to a positive, practical plan for God-honoring friendships. Make the most of opportunities that come when the teenager talks about or struggles with relationships, since these moments are rare. Take the initiative and draw out the teen. Teach him not to be afraid of being honest by being understanding, honestly admitting your own failure, and pointing to the beauty of God's standard and forgiveness.

2. Encourage other parents to be committed to honest, ongoing communication with their teens about sexuality. Parents

need to take responsibility to keep this communication going. Teach parents to be open and unembarrassed, to be willing to invest the time necessary for a robust and honest friendship with their teens. Teach them to ask themselves what *they* are doing specifically to encourage or discourage such a friendship.

3. Always keep the issue of temptation on the table. Know where your teen is being tempted, know how he is dealing with it, and make plans that anticipate temptations to come.

4. Encourage teens to take the long view of relationships. Rather than focus on the joys and pains of the moment, have the teenager start from the perspective of a God-glorifying marriage and work back. What steps need to be taken now, what habits need to be developed now, what things need to be forsaken, to prepare me for God's best? Teach teens to assess their relationships using the sowing and reaping principle in Scripture: The relational seeds they are planting now will result in what kind of harvest?

What is our agenda as we deal with our teenagers and sexuality? We want to be realistic about who they are, realistic about the world they live in, realistic about the contradictory voices they hear, and realistic about our own ambivalence about sex. But we especially want to be sure that our realism reflects the hope of the gospel. This hope is what motivates and shapes our work with teenagers. It is expressed well by the apostle Peter:

> His divine power has given us everything we need for life and godliness through our knowledge of him who called us by his own glory and goodness. Through these he has given us his very great and precious promises, so that through them you may participate in the divine nature and escape the corruption in the world caused by evil desires (2 Peter 1:3–4).

To settle for anything less in the sexual lives of our teenagers is to deny the gospel and to fail in our calling as God's instruments of change in their lives.

Paul David Tripp *is a counselor and faculty member at the Christian Counseling and Educational Foundation in Glenside, Pennsylvania.*

RCL Ministry Booklets

A.D.D.: Wandering Minds and Wired Bodies, by Edward T. Welch

Anger: Escaping the Maze, by David Powlison

Angry at God? Bring Him Your Doubts and Questions, by Robert D. Jones

Bad Memories: Getting Past Your Past, by Robert D. Jones

Depression: The Way Up When You Are Down, by Edward T. Welch

Domestic Abuse: How to Help, by David Powlison, Paul David Tripp, and Edward T. Welch

Forgiveness: "I Just Can't Forgive Myself!" by Robert D. Jones

God's Love: Better than Unconditional, by David Powlison

Guidance: Have I Missed God's Best? by James C. Petty

Homosexuality: Speaking the Truth in Love, by Edward T. Welch

"Just One More": When Desires Don't Take No for an Answer, by Edward T. Welch

Marriage: Whose Dream? by Paul David Tripp

Motives: "Why Do I Do the Things I Do?" by Edward T. Welch

OCD: Freedom for the Obsessive-Compulsive, by Michael R. Emlet

Pornography: Slaying the Dragon, by David Powlison

Pre-Engagement: 5 Questions to Ask Yourselves, by David Powlison and John Yenchko

Priorities: Mastering Time Management, by James C. Petty

Procrastination: First Steps to Change, by Walter Henegar

Self-Injury: When Pain Feels Good, by Edward T. Welch

Sexual Sin: Combatting the Drifting and Cheating, by Jeffrey S. Black

Stress: Peace amid Pressure, by David Powlison

Suffering: Eternity Makes a Difference, by Paul David Tripp

Suicide: Understanding and Intervening by Jeffrey S. Black

Teens and Sex: How Should We Teach Them? by Paul David Tripp

Thankfulness: Even When It Hurts, by Susan Lutz

Why Me? Comfort for the Victimized by David Powlison

Worry: Pursuing a Better Path to Peace, by David Powlison